YOGA
FOR ALL LEVELS

A COMPREHENSIVE GUIDE TO BEST POSES FOR HEALING, RELAXATION, STRENGTH, AND FLEXIBILITY ENHANCEMENT

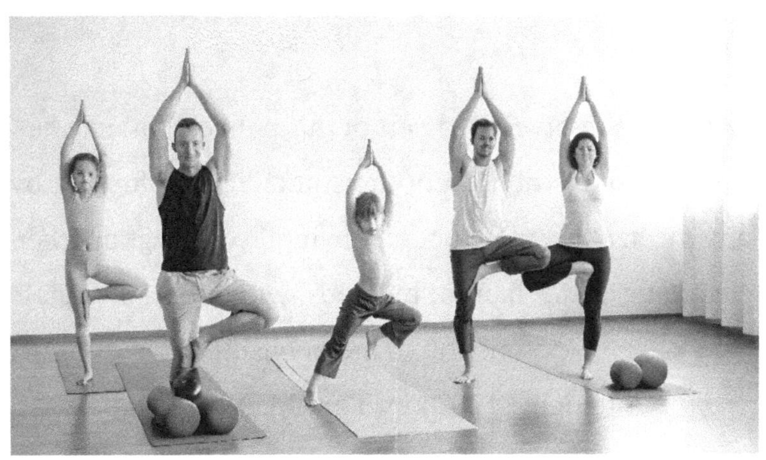

Self-Guided Yoga Practice for Beginners, Intermediates, Juniors and Seniors

Tom M. Yukteswar

TABLE OF CONTENT

Introduction

Unveiling the Depths of Yoga

Purpose and Benefits of Yoga

Why Yoga Is for Everyone

Chapter One: Getting Started with Yoga

How to Warm Up Properly

Creating Your Ideal Yoga Routine

Setting Up Your Yoga Space

Chapter Two: The Physical Benefits of Yoga

Chapter Three: The Mental and Emotional Benefits of Yoga

Chapter Four: Exploring Yoga Poses

Chapter Five: Breathing Techniques in Yoga

Chapter Six: Best Yoga Positions for Warm-up

Chapter Seven: Yoga for Beginners

Chapter Eight: Yoga for Intermediates

Chapter Nine: Yoga for Juniors

Chapter Ten: Yoga for Seniors

Conclusion

Integrating Yoga into Your Daily Life

Continuing Your Yoga Journey

Introduction

Welcome to "Yoga for All Levels," a comprehensive guide to illuminate the transformative power of yoga and empower practitioners of all ages and levels of experience to embark on a journey of self-discovery and self-care.

Unveiling the Depths of Yoga

In the pages of this book, you will discover a treasure trove of wisdom, insights, and practical guidance to help you unlock the full potential of your yoga practice. Whether you are a curious beginner seeking to explore the foundations of yoga or a seasoned practitioner looking to deepen your understanding and refine your technique, "Yoga for All Levels" offers something for everyone.

At its core, yoga is more than just a series of physical postures; it is a holistic system for cultivating health, harmony, and balance in body, mind, and spirit. Through a combination of asanas (poses), pranayama (breath work), and meditation, yoga invites us to explore the interconnectedness of our physical, mental, and emotional selves, fostering a profound sense of integration and wholeness.

One of the most beautiful aspects of yoga is its inclusivity; it is truly a practice for everybody, regardless of age, ability, or background. Whether you are a nimble youngster eager to explore the depths of your flexibility, an elder seeking to maintain vitality and mobility as you age, or anyone in between, "Yoga for All Levels" offers guidance and modifications to meet you exactly where you are on your journey.

So, roll out your mat, take a deep breath, and prepare to embark on a transformative journey of self-discovery and self-care. Within the pages of "Yoga for All Levels," you will find everything you need to cultivate strength, flexibility, relaxation, and healing in body, mind, and spirit. Whether you have five minutes or fifty, whether you are practicing in the comfort of your living room or amidst the beauty of nature, the transformative power of yoga awaits you.

Purpose and Benefits of Yoga

Envision a weary traveler, burdened by the weight of their worldly cares, stumbling upon an oasis in the midst of a scorching desert. As they sink into the cool shade of towering palms, a sense of profound relief washes over them, and they realize that this sanctuary offers more than just physical respite—it is a sanctuary for the soul. Similarly, yoga presents us with an oasis of stillness amidst the ceaseless demands of our daily lives, inviting us to journey inward and discover the boundless wellspring of peace that resides within.

"Yoga is the journey of the self, through the self, to the self." These profound words from the Bhagavad Gita encapsulate the essence of yoga, reminding us that its true purpose extends far beyond the physical postures we practice on the mat. At its core, yoga is a path of self-discovery, a journey that leads us back to the essence of who we are and the interconnectedness of all things.

Picture a tranquil mountain lake, nestled amidst a pristine alpine landscape. Its surface is as smooth as glass, reflecting the majestic peaks that loom overhead. Despite the tumultuous storms that may rage above, the lake remains undisturbed, a symbol of unwavering serenity. In much the same way, yoga empowers us to cultivate a sense of inner calm amidst the turbulence of life. Through the practice of mindfulness, breath work, and movement, we learn to anchor ourselves in the present moment, finding solace and clarity amidst the chaos.

In the pages that follow, we will embark on a journey of exploration and self-discovery, delving into the transformative power of yoga to heal the body, soothe the mind, and nourish the soul. Whether you are a seasoned practitioner or a curious newcomer, "Yoga for All Levels" offers a wealth of wisdom and guidance to support you on your path to greater health, happiness, and harmony.

Why Yoga Is for Everyone

In a world where physical fitness trends come and go, yoga stands apart as a timeless practice accessible to all. Regardless of age, body type, or fitness level, yoga offers a myriad of benefits that extend far beyond the physical realm. Here's why yoga truly is for everyone:

1. Adaptability: One of the most beautiful aspects of yoga is its adaptability. Whether you're a beginner or an experienced practitioner, yoga can be tailored to meet you exactly where you are on your journey. With modifications and variations available for every pose, individuals of all abilities can participate and experience the benefits of yoga.

2. Inclusivity: Unlike many fitness practices that prioritize certain body types or levels of athleticism, yoga embraces diversity and inclusivity. There is no one-size-fits-all approach to yoga, and practitioners come in all shapes, sizes, and backgrounds. Regardless of age, gender, or physical condition, everyone can find a place in the yoga community.

3. Mind-Body Connection: Yoga is not just about physical exercise; it's about cultivating a deep connection between mind, body, and spirit. Through the practice of asanas (poses), pranayama (breath work), and meditation, yoga encourages individuals to tune into their bodies, quiet their minds, and cultivate inner peace and self-awareness.

4. Stress Relief: In today's fast-paced world, stress has become a pervasive issue affecting people of all ages. Yoga offers a powerful antidote to stress, helping individuals to release tension, quiet the mind, and find a sense of calm amidst the chaos. By incorporating mindfulness and relaxation techniques, yoga equips practitioners with valuable tools for managing stress and promoting emotional well-being.

5. **Physical Benefits:** While yoga is often celebrated for its mental and emotional benefits, it also offers a wide range of physical benefits. From improving flexibility and strength to promoting better posture and balance, yoga supports overall physical health and vitality. Whether you're looking to tone muscles, increase mobility, or prevent injury, yoga offers a comprehensive workout for the body.

6. **Lifelong Practice:** Unlike many forms of exercise that may become challenging or inaccessible as we age, yoga is a practice that can be sustained throughout the lifespan. Whether you're in your teens or your golden years, yoga offers a gentle and sustainable way to stay active, healthy, and vibrant at every stage of life.

Chapter One:
Getting Started with Yoga

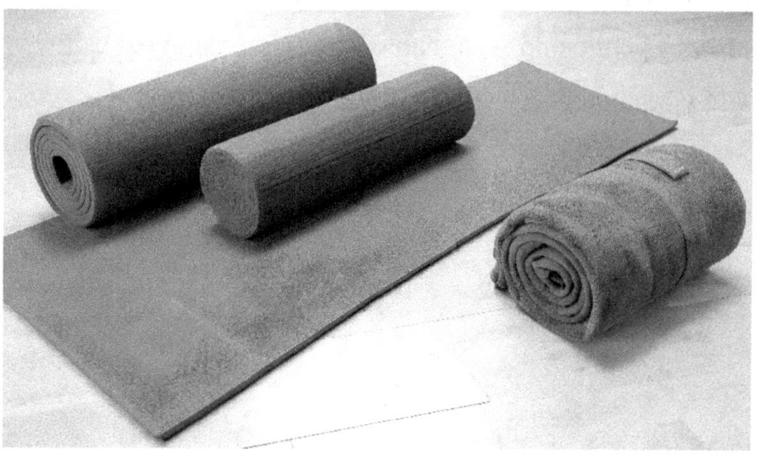

Embarking on a yoga journey can be both exhilarating and intimidating, especially if you're new to the practice. In this chapter, you will be guide through the essential steps to help you begin your yoga practice with confidence and ease.

1. Setting Intentions

Before diving into your first yoga session, take a moment to set your intentions. What do you hope to gain from your practice? Whether it's increased flexibility, stress relief, or simply a sense of well-being, clarifying your intentions will help you stay focused and motivated throughout your journey.

2. Creating Your Sacred Space

Find a quiet, clutter-free space where you can practice without distractions. Set up your yoga mat and any props you may need; such as blocks or straps. Consider adding elements that inspire tranquility, such as candles, incense, or soothing music. Creating a sacred space will enhance your practice and deepen your connection to the present moment.

3. Cultivating Mindfulness

Yoga is not just about physical postures; it's also about cultivating mindfulness and awareness. Before beginning your practice, take a few moments to center yourself. Close your eyes, connect with your breath, and tune into the sensations of your body. Allow yourself to let go of any distractions or worries, and simply be present with yourself on the mat.

4. Starting with the Basics

If you're new to yoga, it's essential to start with the basics. Begin with gentle, beginner-friendly poses that focus on building strength, flexibility, and body awareness. Pay attention to proper alignment and listen to your body's signals. Remember that yoga is a journey, not a destination, so be patient and compassionate with yourself as you learn and grow.

5. Exploring Different Styles

Yoga is a diverse practice with many different styles and approaches. Take the time to explore different styles of yoga, such as Hatha, Vinyasa, or Yin, to find what resonates with you. Each style offers unique benefits and challenges, so don't be afraid to step out of your comfort zone and try something new.

6. Practicing Consistency

Consistency is key to reaping the full benefits of yoga. Aim to practice regularly, even if it's just for a few minutes each day. Consistency will help you build strength, flexibility, and mindfulness over time, allowing you to experience greater progress and transformation in your practice.

7. Embracing the Journey

Above all, remember that yoga is a journey, not a destination. Embrace the ups and downs, the challenges and triumphs, and allow yourself to grow and evolve along the way. Stay open-minded, curious, and compassionate towards yourself and others as you explore the vast and beautiful world of yoga.

In the following chapters, we'll delve deeper into specific aspects of yoga practice, including breath work, meditation, and advanced poses. But for now, take these foundational steps to heart as you begin your yoga journey. With dedication, patience, and an open heart, you'll discover the profound joy and transformation that yoga has to offer.

How to Warm Up Properly

Warming up before engaging in any physical activity is essential to prepare the body for movement, prevent injury, and optimize performance. In the context of yoga, a proper warm-up not only loosens tight muscles and joints but also helps to center the mind and cultivate presence before diving into the more intensive aspects of the practice. Here are some effective strategies for warming up properly in preparation for your yoga practice:

1. Mindful Breathing: Begin by finding a comfortable seated position on your mat. Close your eyes and take a few moments to connect with your breath. Inhale deeply through your nose, feeling the breath expand your lungs and fill your belly. Exhale fully, releasing any tension or distractions from your mind. Continue this deep, mindful breathing for several rounds, allowing yourself to arrive fully in the present moment.

2. Gentle Movement: Gradually introduce gentle movements to awaken the body and increase circulation.

Start with slow neck rolls, gently rotating your head in a circular motion to release tension in the neck and shoulders. Then, move on to shoulder rolls, rolling your shoulders forward and backward in smooth, controlled movements. Explore gentle twists, side stretches, and forward folds to loosen the spine and increase mobility in the torso.

3. Dynamic Stretching: Incorporate dynamic stretches to lengthen and warm up the major muscle groups of the body. Perform dynamic lunges, stepping forward with one foot and lowering your hips into a lunge position, then switching to the other side. Flow through a series of Sun Salutations, linking breath with movement as you transition between poses such as Downward-Facing Dog, Plank, and Cobra or Upward-Facing Dog.

4. Joint Mobilization: Pay attention to the joints, gently moving them through their full range of motion to lubricate the joints and improve mobility. Perform wrist circles, ankle circles, and knee circles to warm up the wrists, ankles, and knees respectively. Incorporate gentle movements such as wrist flexion and extension, ankle circles, and knee lifts to prepare these joints for the demands of your yoga practice.

5. Centering Meditation: Conclude your warm-up with a brief centering meditation to ground yourself and set a positive intention for your practice. Sit or lie down comfortably on your mat, close your eyes, and bring your awareness to your breath. Take a few moments to cultivate a sense of inner calm and focus, allowing any lingering tension or distractions to melt away.

By incorporating these elements into your warm-up routine, you can effectively prepare your body, mind, and spirit for the transformative journey that lies ahead on your yoga mat. Remember to listen to your body, honor its needs, and approach your practice with patience, mindfulness, and compassion. With a proper warm-up, you can lay the foundation for a safe, enjoyable, and deeply fulfilling yoga experience.

Creating Your Ideal Yoga Routine

Crafting your ideal yoga routine is akin to designing a personalized roadmap to well-being, tailored to your unique needs, preferences, and goals. Whether you're seeking to cultivate strength and flexibility, alleviate stress and tension, or simply find moments of peace and tranquility amidst the chaos of daily life, a thoughtfully curated yoga practice can serve as a sanctuary for body, mind, and spirit. Here's how to create a yoga routine that resonates with you:

1. Define Your Objectives: Begin by clarifying your intentions and objectives for your yoga practice. Are you looking to build strength and endurance? Enhance flexibility and mobility? Reduce stress and promote relaxation? Identifying your goals will guide the structure and focus of your routine.

2. Assess Your Schedule: Consider your daily commitments, time constraints, and energy levels when designing your yoga routine. Aim to carve out dedicated time for practice, whether it's a brief session in the morning to energize your day or a longer session in the evening to unwind and release tension.

3. Select Your Practices: Choose a combination of asanas (poses), pranayama (breathwork), and meditation techniques that align with your objectives and preferences. Mix and match different styles and intensity levels to create a well-rounded practice that addresses your physical, mental, and emotional needs.

4. Establish a Structure: Structure your yoga routine in a way that flows seamlessly from one component to the next, creating a harmonious and balanced practice. Begin with a gentle warm-up to prepare your body and mind for movement, followed by a series of dynamic asanas to build strength and flexibility. Incorporate breathwork and mindfulness practices to cultivate presence and awareness, and conclude with a soothing cool-down and relaxation to integrate the benefits of your practice.

5. Listen to Your Body: Pay attention to the signals and sensations that arise within your body during your yoga practice. Honor your limits and boundaries, modifying poses and intensity levels as needed to ensure safety and comfort. Cultivate a compassionate and non-judgmental attitude towards yourself, embracing the journey of self-discovery and self-care with patience and kindness.

6. Experiment and Adapt: Be open to experimentation and adaptation as you refine your yoga routine over time. Explore new poses, techniques, and sequences, and adjust your practice according to feedback from your body and mind. Stay curious and receptive to the ever-evolving nature of your yoga journey.

7. Consistency is Key: Establishing a consistent yoga routine is essential for reaping the full benefits of your practice. Commit to showing up on your mat regularly, even on days when motivation may wane or obstacles arise. Remember that every moment of practice is an opportunity for growth, transformation, and self-discovery.

By creating and committing to your ideal yoga routine, you embark on a journey of self-care, self-discovery, and holistic well-being that has the power to enrich every aspect of your life. Embrace the process with curiosity, compassion, and dedication, and allow your practice to unfold organically, nourishing body, mind, and spirit with each breath and movement.

Setting Up Your Yoga Space

Creating a dedicated yoga space in your home can significantly enhance the quality of your practice and deepen your connection to the ancient tradition of yoga. Whether you have a spacious room to devote entirely to yoga or just a small corner of your living space, here are some tips for setting up a nurturing and inspiring environment for your practice:

1. Choose a Quiet and Clutter-Free Area: Select a space in your home that is free from distractions and clutter. Ideally, this area should be quiet and peaceful, allowing you to immerse yourself fully in your practice without external disturbances.

2. Clear the Space: Before you begin practicing yoga in your chosen area, take a few moments to clear away any clutter or unnecessary items. Create a clean and inviting environment that will help you feel calm and focused.

3. Consider Lighting: Natural light can be a wonderful addition to your yoga space, as it creates a sense of warmth and openness. If possible, position your mat near a window where you can enjoy the soft glow of sunlight streaming in. Alternatively, you can use lamps or candles to create a cozy atmosphere during evening practices.

4. Add Personal Touches: Infuse your yoga space with elements that inspire and uplift you. This could include plants, inspirational quotes or artwork, crystals, or any other items that hold special meaning for you. Surrounding yourself with objects that evoke feelings of joy, peace, and beauty can enhance your overall experience of yoga.

5. Invest in Essential Equipment: While you don't need a lot of fancy equipment to practice yoga, there are a few key items that can enhance your comfort and support during your practice. Consider investing in a high-quality yoga mat, props such as blocks and straps, and a comfortable cushion or bolster for meditation and relaxation.

6. Create Ambiance: Set the mood for your practice by incorporating elements that engage your senses. Play soothing music or nature sounds to create a calming atmosphere, use essential oils or incense to evoke feelings of relaxation, and consider dimming the lights or lighting candles to enhance the sense of tranquility.

7. Maintain Cleanliness: Keep your yoga space clean and tidy to promote a sense of well-being and harmony. Regularly dust and vacuum the area, and wash your yoga mat and props as needed to ensure they remain fresh and hygienic.

By taking the time to thoughtfully design and set up your yoga space, you can create a sacred sanctuary where you can retreat to nourish your body, mind, and spirit through the practice of yoga. Whether you are embarking on a solo practice or sharing the space with loved ones, cultivating a dedicated yoga space can support you in deepening your connection to yourself and to the ancient tradition of yoga.

Chapter Two:

The Physical Benefits of Yoga

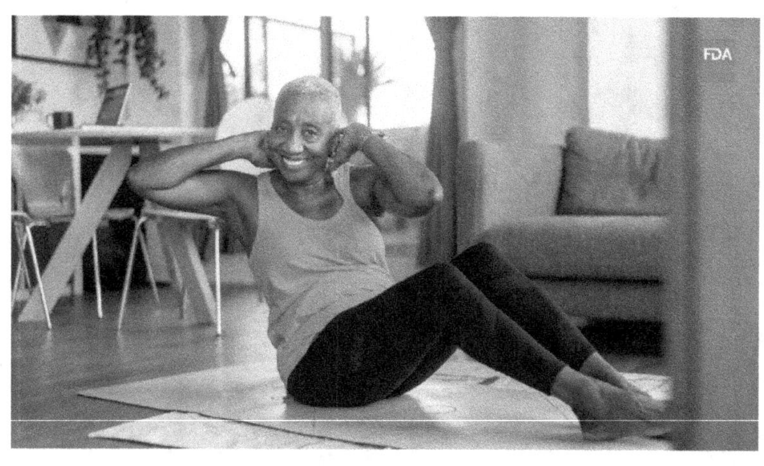

In this chapter, we will delve into the myriad ways in which the practice of yoga can positively impact our physical well-being. From increasing strength and flexibility to relieving pain and preventing injury, yoga offers a holistic approach to fitness that encompasses both the body and the mind.

1. Increasing Strength and Flexibility

Yoga is renowned for its ability to build strength and enhance flexibility in a balanced and sustainable manner. Through a combination of dynamic movements, static holds, and isometric contractions, yoga poses target and engage muscles throughout the entire body, helping to develop functional strength and improve range of motion. As we cultivate greater strength and flexibility through our yoga practice, we not only enhance our physical capabilities but also foster a deeper sense of connection and awareness within ourselves.

2. Relieving Pain and Preventing Injury

One of the most compelling benefits of yoga is its potential to alleviate chronic pain and reduce the risk of injury. By improving posture, alignment, and body awareness, yoga helps to correct imbalances and alleviate tension in the muscles and joints, thereby reducing the likelihood of strain and injury. Additionally, many yoga poses are specifically designed to target common areas of discomfort, such as the lower back, hips, and shoulders, offering gentle yet effective relief from pain and stiffness.

3. Developing Strong and Healthy Bones, Muscles, Joints, and Ligaments

Regular practice of yoga can also contribute to the development of strong and resilient bones, muscles, joints, and ligaments. Weight-bearing poses such as standing balances and arm balances help to stimulate bone density and promote skeletal health, reducing the risk of osteoporosis and age-related bone loss. Meanwhile, dynamic movements and gentle stretches improve joint mobility and lubrication, supporting overall joint health and longevity. By nurturing the structural integrity of our bodies through yoga, we can enjoy greater stability, mobility, and vitality as we age.

4. Enhancing Athletic Performance

For athletes and fitness enthusiasts, yoga can serve as a valuable complement to traditional training regimens, helping to improve performance, prevent injuries, and promote recovery. By enhancing flexibility, mobility, and body awareness, yoga can optimize biomechanics and movement efficiency, allowing athletes to move more freely and fluidly in their chosen sport or activity. Additionally, the focus on breath control and mental focus in yoga can help athletes cultivate greater concentration, resilience, and mental clarity, enabling them to perform at their peak, both on and off the field.

Chapter Three:
The Mental and Emotional Benefits of Yoga

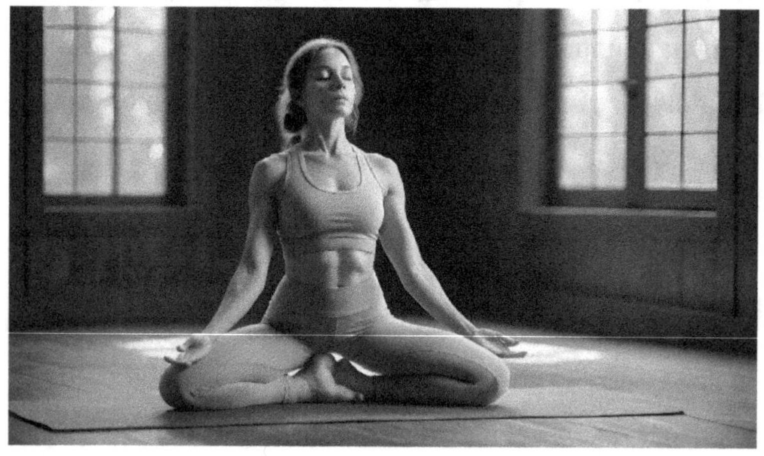

In the fast-paced world we live in, where stress, anxiety, and emotional turbulence are all too common, yoga emerges as a powerful tool for cultivating mental and emotional well-being. In this chapter, we will explore the profound ways in which a regular yoga practice can support and enhance our mental and emotional health, fostering greater peace, clarity, and resilience in the face of life's challenges.

1. Reducing Stress and Anxiety

Yoga offers a sanctuary of calm amidst the chaos of our daily lives. Through a combination of mindful movement, breath awareness, and relaxation techniques, yoga has been shown to significantly reduce levels of stress and anxiety. By tuning into the present moment and releasing tension from the body and mind, we can cultivate a deep sense of relaxation and tranquility that permeates every aspect of our lives.

2. Enhancing Mental Clarity and Focus

The practice of yoga encourages us to cultivate a state of mindful awareness, allowing us to quiet the chatter of the mind and focus our attention on the present moment. Through the coordination of breath and movement, we learn to synchronize mind and body, sharpening our mental faculties and enhancing our ability to concentrate and focus. This heightened sense of mental clarity can extend beyond the yoga mat, empowering us to approach tasks and challenges with greater efficiency and effectiveness.

3. Cultivating Emotional Resilience

Life is full of ups and downs, joys and sorrows, triumphs and setbacks. Yoga teaches us to navigate the ever-changing landscape of our emotions with grace and resilience. By cultivating self-awareness and compassion through the practice of yoga, we can learn to observe our thoughts and feelings without judgment, allowing them to arise and pass away like waves on the ocean. In doing so, we develop the inner strength and resilience to weather life's storms with equanimity and grace.

4. Fostering Self-Compassion and Acceptance

Yoga invites us to cultivate a deep sense of self-compassion and acceptance, embracing ourselves exactly as we are in this moment. Through the practice of yoga, we learn to listen to our bodies, honor our limitations, and celebrate our strengths. By cultivating a sense of loving-kindness towards ourselves, we can release the burden of self-criticism and perfectionism, allowing ourselves to embrace our inherent worthiness and embrace the fullness of our humanity.

Chapter Four:
Exploring Yoga Poses

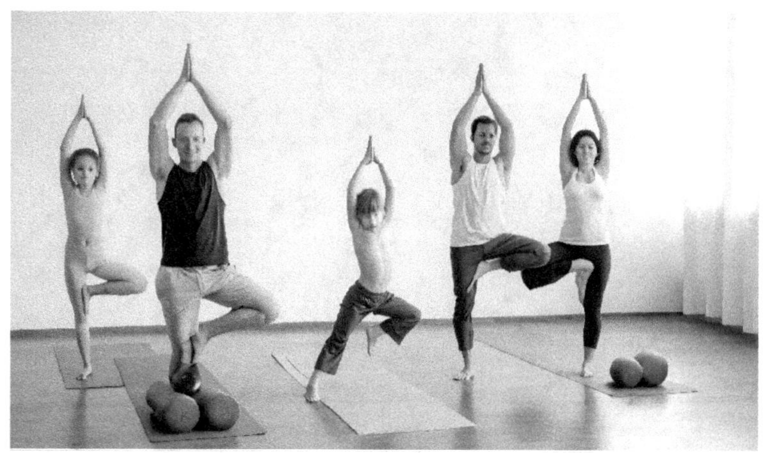

In the vast landscape of yoga, the exploration of poses is akin to embarking on a journey of self-discovery and physical embodiment. Each pose, or asana, offers a unique opportunity to connect with our bodies, cultivate strength and flexibility, and foster a sense of inner peace and harmony. In this chapter, we will delve into the rich tapestry of yoga poses, exploring proper technique, modifications for different levels of experience, and the specific benefits each pose offers.

Understanding Proper Technique

Proper technique is essential for safely and effectively practicing yoga poses. Throughout this chapter, we will provide detailed instructions and demonstrations to guide you in executing each pose with precision and mindfulness. From the alignment of your body to the engagement of your muscles and the rhythm of your breath, we will explore how to approach each pose with intention and awareness.

Modifications for Different Levels of Experience

Yoga is a practice that is accessible to people of all ages, abilities, and levels of experience. Whether you are brand new to yoga or have been practicing for years, there are modifications and variations of poses that can be tailored to suit your individual needs and goals. In this chapter, we will offer modifications for beginners who may be working to build strength and flexibility, as well as variations for more experienced practitioners looking to deepen their practice.

Specific Benefits of Each Pose

Each yoga pose offers a unique set of benefits for the body, mind, and spirit. From improving strength and flexibility to reducing stress and promoting relaxation, the benefits of yoga poses are as diverse as the poses themselves. Throughout this chapter, we will explore the specific benefits of each pose, helping you to understand how they can support your overall health and well-being.

Embarking on Your Pose Exploration

As you journey through this chapter, we encourage you to approach the exploration of yoga poses with an open mind and a sense of curiosity. Allow yourself to be present in each moment, tuning in to the sensations in your body and the rhythms of your breath. Whether you are practicing in the comfort of your own home, in a studio surrounded by fellow yogis, or outdoors amidst the beauty of nature, let each pose be an opportunity to connect with yourself on a deeper level and to cultivate a greater sense of balance, vitality, and joy.

Chapter Five:
Breathing Techniques in Yoga

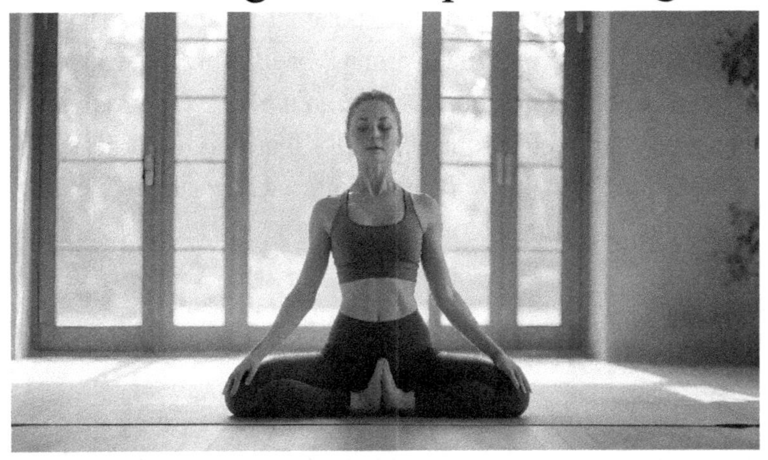

In the practice of yoga, breath is the vital thread that weaves together body, mind, and spirit. Chapter 6 of "Yoga for All Levels" delves into the profound significance of breath in the practice of yoga and introduces a variety of breathing techniques to enhance your overall well-being and deepen your connection to the present moment.

The Importance of Breath

Breath is the bridge between the outer world and our inner landscape, serving as a powerful tool for cultivating awareness, presence, and inner peace. In yoga philosophy, the breath is referred to as "prana," or life force energy, and is believed to be the vehicle through which we nourish and energize every cell of our being. By learning to harness the power of the breath, we can tap into a wellspring of vitality, clarity, and serenity.

The Role of Breath in Yoga Practice

In the practice of yoga, breath serves as the guiding force that informs our movement, anchors our awareness, and invites us to cultivate a deep sense of mindfulness. Each inhale invites expansion and receptivity, while each exhale offers release and surrender, creating a seamless flow of energy throughout the body. By synchronizing breath with movement, we can move with greater grace, ease, and intention, allowing the practice to unfold with a sense of fluidity and grace.

Exploring Breathing Techniques

Chapter 6 offers a comprehensive exploration of various breathing techniques, each designed to serve a specific purpose and enhance your yoga practice. From calming and centering breaths to invigorating and energizing techniques, you will learn how to tailor your breath to support your unique needs and intentions on the mat. Whether you are seeking to cultivate inner peace, build strength and stamina, or deepen your meditation practice, there is a breath technique to guide you on your journey.

Guided Practices

Throughout this chapter, you will find guided practices and step-by-step instructions to help you incorporate breathing techniques into your yoga practice. Whether you are a beginner or an experienced practitioner, these accessible exercises will empower you to tap into the transformative power of breath and cultivate a greater sense of presence and vitality in your practice and in your life.

Embrace the Power of Breath!

Chapter Six:
Best Yoga Positions
for Warm-up

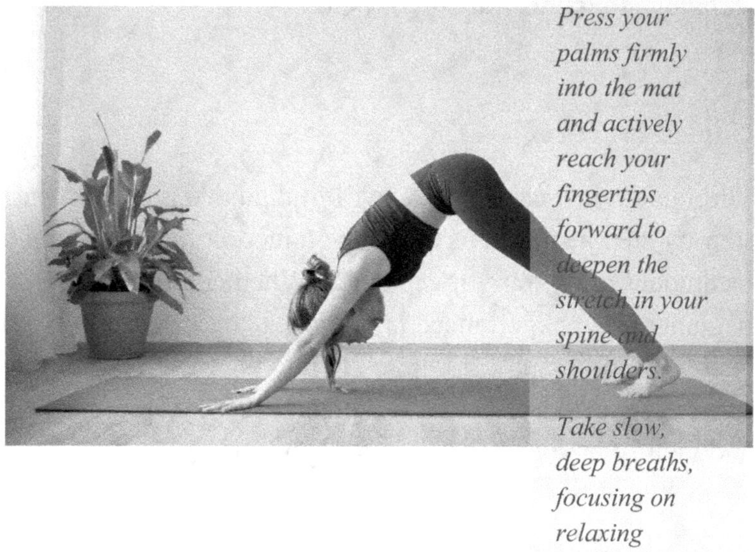

1. Child's Pose (Balasana)

Description:

1. Begin by kneeling on the mat with your big toes
    touching and knees spread apart.

2. Sit back on your heels and extend your arms forward, lowering your torso between your thighs.

3. Rest your forehead on the mat and relax your entire body.

- Beginners: 1-2 minutes
- Intermediates: 2-3 minutes;
- Juniors: 3-4 minutes
- Seniors: 4-5 minutes

Move slowly and mindfully, coordinating each movement with your breath.

Focus on articulating each vertebra as you move between Cat and Cow Poses.

Benefits:

Child's Pose gently stretches the spine, hips, thighs, and ankles, while promoting relaxation and relieving stress and fatigue.

2. Cat-Cow Pose (Marjaryasana-Bitilasana)

Description:

1. Start on your hands and knees, with wrists directly under shoulders and knees under hips.

2. Inhale, arch your back, lift your tailbone and chest toward the ceiling (Cow Pose).

3. Exhale, round your spine, tuck your chin to your chest, and draw your belly button towards your spine (Cat Pose).

- Beginners: 1-2 minutes
- Intermediates: 2-3 minutes
- Juniors: 3-4 minutes
- Seniors: 4-5 minutes.

Benefits:

Cat-Cow Pose helps to warm up the spine, improve spinal flexibility, and increase circulation to the spinal discs. It also massages the internal organs and promotes healthy digestion.

Tips:

Keep a slight bend in your knees if your hamstrings feel tight.

Spread your fingers wide and press firmly into the mat to distribute weight evenly.

Engage your core muscles and relax your neck.

3. Downward-Facing Dog Pose (Adho Mukha Svanasana)

Description:

1. Start on your hands and knees, tuck your toes, and lift your hips up and back,
2. forming an inverted V shape with your body.
3. Keep your hands shoulder-width apart and feet hip-width apart.
4. Press your palms into the mat and lengthen your spine.

- Beginners: 30 seconds to 1 minute
- Intermediates: 1-2 minutes
- Juniors: 2-3 minutes
- Seniors: 3-4 minutes.

Benefits:

Downward-Facing Dog stretches the entire body, particularly the shoulders, hamstrings, calves, and spine. It also strengthens the arms and legs, improves circulation, and calms the mind.

4. Standing Forward Fold (Uttanasana

Description:

1. Stand tall with feet hip-width apart.
2. Exhale, hinge at the hips, and fold forward, bringing your hands to the floor or grabbing opposite elbows.
3. Let your head hang heavy and relax your neck

Tips:

Keep a slight bend in your knees to protect the hamstrings.

If your hands don't reach the floor, place them on blocks or your shins.

Relax your shoulders away from your ears and breathe deeply into your hamstrings.

- Beginners: 30 seconds to 1 minute
- Intermediates: 1-2 minutes
- Juniors: 2-3 minutes
- Seniors: 3-4 minutes.

Benefits:

Standing Forward Fold stretches the hamstrings, calves, and hips, while also releasing tension in the spine and shoulders. It improves flexibility, calms the mind, and relieves stress and anxiety.

5. Seated Forward Bend (Paschimottanasana)

Description:

1. Sit on the mat with legs extended in front of you. Inhale, lengthen your spine, and exhale, hinge at the hips to fold forward, reaching for your feet or shins.
2. Keep your spine long and avoid rounding your back.

- Beginners: 30 seconds to 1 minute
- Intermediates: 1-2 minutes
- Juniors: 2-3 minutes
- Seniors: 3-4 minutes.

Benefits:

Seated Forward Bend stretches the entire back body, including the spine, hamstrings, and calves. It stimulates the abdominal organs, improves digestion, and soothes the nervous system.

6. Downward-Facing Dog (Adho Mukha Svanasana)

Description:

1. Begin on your hands and knees, then lift your hips up towards the ceiling, coming into an inverted V shape.
2. Press your hands firmly into the mat, with your fingers spread wide apart.
3. Keep your heels reaching towards the ground and your head relaxed between your arms.

- Beginners: 30 seconds - 1 minute
- Intermediates: 1-2 minutes
- Juniors: 2-3 minutes
- Seniors: 3-4 minutes

Benefits:

Downward-Facing Dog stretches the entire body, including the shoulders, hamstrings, calves, and spine. It also strengthens the arms, shoulders, and core muscles, improves circulation, and energizes the body.

7. Standing Forward Bend (Uttanasana)

Description:

1. Stand tall with your feet hip-width apart.
2. Inhale as you lengthen your spine, then exhale as you hinge at the hips and fold forward, bringing your chest towards your thighs and your hands towards the ground or your shins.

- Beginners: 30 seconds - 1 minute,
- Intermediates: 1-2 minutes,
- Juniors: 2-3 minutes,
- Seniors: 3-4 minutes

Benefits:

Standing Forward Bend stretches the entire back side of the body, including the hamstrings, calves, spine, and shoulders. It also calms the mind, relieves stress and anxiety, and improves digestion.

8. Mountain Pose (Tadasana)

Description:

1. Stand tall with your feet hip-width apart, arms by your sides, and palms facing forward.
2. Engage your thighs, lift your chest, and roll your shoulders back.
3. Relax your face and breathe deeply.

Tips:

Ground down through your feet, imagining roots growing from the soles.

Lengthen through the crown of your head.

Keep your gaze soft and steady.

- Beginners: 1-2 minutes,
- Intermediates: 2-3 minutes,
- Juniors: 3-4 minutes,
- Seniors: 1-2 minutes

Benefits:

Improves posture, strengthens thighs and core, increases body awareness.

9. Sun Salutation (Surya Namaskar)

Description:

1. A sequence of poses performed in a flowing sequence.
2. Begin in Mountain Pose, inhale, raise arms overhead, exhale, fold forward, inhale, lift halfway, exhale, step or jump back to Plank Pose,
3. Lower down to Chaturanga Dandasana, inhale, upward-facing dog, exhale, return to Mountain Pose.

- Beginners: 3-5 rounds,
  Intermediates: 5-8 rounds,
- Juniors: 8-10 rounds,
- Seniors: 3-5 rounds

Benefits:

Full body warm-up, improves circulation, boosts energy levels.

10. Garland Pose (Malasana)

Description:

1. Begin in a squat position with your feet slightly wider than hip-width apart, toes turned out.
2. Lower your hips towards the floor, keeping your heels on the ground.
3. Bring your palms together at your heart center and use your elbows to press your knees gently open.

Tips:

If your heels lift off the ground, place a folded blanket or block under them for support.

Keep your spine long and chest lifted to avoid rounding forward.

Press your elbows into your knees to deepen the stretch in the hips.

- Beginners: 1 -2 minute
- Intermediates: 1-2 minutes
- Juniors: 1-3 minutes
- Seniors: 3-4 minutes.

Benefits:

Opens the hips, groin, and inner thighs, strengthens the legs, ankles, and feet, improves mobility and flexibility in the lower body.

Chapter Seven:
Yoga for Beginners

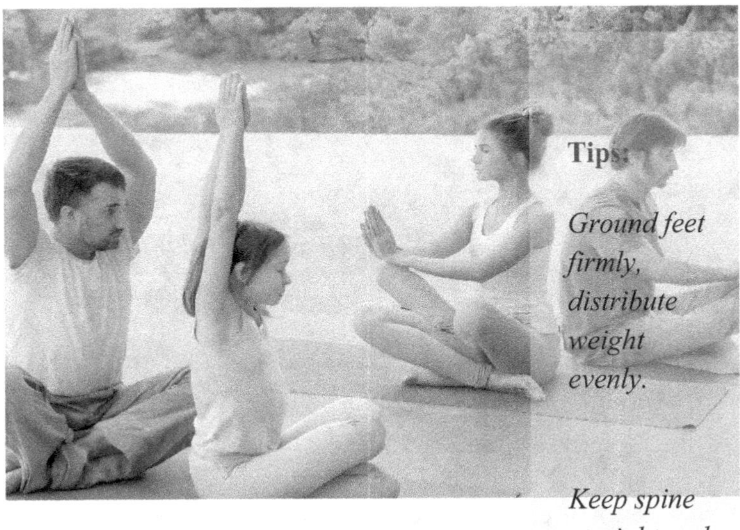

1. Mountain Pose (Tadasana)

Description:

1. Stand tall with feet together, arms by your sides, palms facing forward.

2. Engage thighs, lift chest, and roll shoulders back. Relax face and breathe deeply.

- Duration: 1-2 minutes

Benefits:

Improves posture, strengthens legs, increases body awareness.

2. Downward-Facing Dog (Adho Mukha Svanasana)

Description:

1. Start on hands and knees, tuck toes under, lift hips up and back, forming an inverted V-shape.

2. Hands shoulder-width apart, feet hip-width apart, heels reaching towards the ground

- Duration: 1-2 minutes

Benefits:

Stretches hamstrings, calves, and shoulders, strengthens arms and legs, relieves stress.

3. Child's Pose (Balasana)

Description:

1. Kneel on the mat, big toes touching, knees apart.
2. Lower torso between thighs, extend arms forward with palms down, and rest forehead on the mat.

Tips:

Relax shoulders, breathe deeply into the back, and sink hips towards heels.

Use a cushion under forehead or knees if needed.

- Duration: 1-2 minutes

Benefits:

Stretches hips, thighs, and ankles, releases tension in back and shoulders, calms the mind.

4. Cat-Cow Pose (Marjaryasana-Bitilasana)

Description:

1. Start on hands and knees, wrists under shoulders, knees under hips. Inhale, arch back and lift tailbone/head (Cow Pose), exhale, round spine and tuck chin (Cat Pose).

2. Flow between the two poses with breath.

- Duration: 1-2 minutes

Benefits:

Warms up spine, massages internal organs, improves spinal flexibility.

5. Warrior I (Virabhadrasana I)

Description:

1. From Downward-Facing Dog, step right foot forward between hands, aligning knee over ankle.

2. Spin back foot flat on the mat at a 45-degree angle, square hips forward, and reach arms overhead.

Tips:

Keep front knee bent at 90 degrees, press back heel into the ground, and lift torso away from thighs.

Engage core muscles for stability.

- Duration: 30 seconds to 1 minute per side

Benefits:

Strengthens legs, opens hips, chest, and shoulders, builds focus and determination.

6. Warrior II (Virabhadrasana II)

Description:

1. From Warrior I, open hips and arms to the sides, parallel to the mat.

2. Front heel aligns with back arch, gaze over front fingertips.

- Duration: 30 seconds to 1 minute per side

Benefits:

Improves concentration, builds stamina, stretches groins and hips.

7. Triangle Pose (Trikonasana)

Description:

1. From Warrior II, straighten front leg, reach forward with front hand, and hinge at the hip to lower hand to shin, ankle, or floor.

2. Extend top arm towards the ceiling, gaze up or down.

Tips:

Keep legs straight but not locked, engage core muscles for stability, and lengthen spine.

Use a block under bottom hand if unable to reach the floor.

- Duration: 30 seconds to 1 minute per side

Benefits:

Stretches hamstrings, groins, and hips, improves balance and stability, stimulates abdominal organs.

8. Bridge Pose (Setu Bandhasana)

Description:

1. Lie on back, knees bent, feet hip-width apart and flat on the mat.

2. Press feet into the ground, lift hips towards the ceiling, interlace fingers under the back and roll shoulders under.

- Duration: 30 seconds to 1 minute

Benefits:

Strengthens back, glutes, and thighs, opens chest and shoulders, improves spine flexibility.

9. Corpse Pose (Savasana)

Description:

1. Lie on back, arms by sides, palms facing up, feet relaxed and falling out to the sides.

2. Close eyes, relax entire body, and focus on deep, even breaths.

Tips:

Release all tension from the body, surrender to the support of the earth beneath you, and allow the mind to become still.

- Duration: 30 seconds to 1 minute

Benefits:

Relaxes body and mind, reduces stress and anxiety, promotes deep relaxation and rejuvenation.

10. Seated Forward Bend (Paschimottanasana)

Description:

1. Sit on the mat with legs extended forward.

2. Inhale, lengthen spine, exhale, hinge at hips and fold forward, reaching for feet or shins.

- Duration: 30 seconds to 1 minute

Benefits:

Stretches spine, hamstrings, and calves, calms the mind, stimulates abdominal organs.

11. Easy Pose (Sukhasana)

Description:

1. Sit on the mat with legs crossed, shins stacked, and feet under opposite knees.

2. Place hands on knees or in prayer position.

- Duration: 1-2 minute

Benefits:

Opens hips and groin, improves posture, calms the mind.

Ground sit bones, lengthen spine with each inhale, deepen twist with each exhale.

Option to hug right knee with left arm for deeper stretch.

12. Seated Spinal Twist (Ardha Matsyendrasana)

Description:

1. Sit on the mat with legs extended, bend right knee, place foot outside left knee.

2. Inhale, lengthen spine, exhale, twist torso to the right, placing left elbow outside right knee.

- Duration: 30 seconds to 1 minute

Benefits:

Increases spinal mobility, massages abdominal organs, improves digestion.

13. Legs-Up-the-Wall Pose (Viparita Karani)

Description:

1. Sit close to a wall, lie on back, extend legs up the wall with heels resting against it.

2. Arms by sides, palms facing up, and close eyes.

Tips:

Keep legs straight or slightly bent, relax entire body, and focus on deep belly breathing.

Use a folded blanket under hips for support if needed.

- Duration: 3-5 minutes

Benefits:

Relieves tired legs and feet, reduces swelling, promotes relaxation and stress relief.

14. Cobra Pose (Bhujangasana)

Description:

1. Lie on stomach, legs together, hands under shoulders, elbows close to body.

2. Inhale, press into palms, lift chest and head off the mat, keeping shoulders down.

Tips:

Engage back muscles, lengthen spine, and draw shoulder blades together.

Keep elbows close to body, avoid locking elbows.

- Duration: 15-30 seconds

Benefits:

Strengthens spine, opens chest and shoulders, improves posture.

15. Seated Forward Bend (Paschimottanasana)

Description:

1. Sit on the mat with legs extended forward.

2. Inhale, lengthen spine, exhale, hinge at hips and fold forward, reaching for feet or shins.

- Duration: 30 seconds to 1 minute

Benefits:

Stretches spine, hamstrings, and calves, calms the mind, stimulates abdominal organs.

Chapter Eight:
Yoga for Intermediates

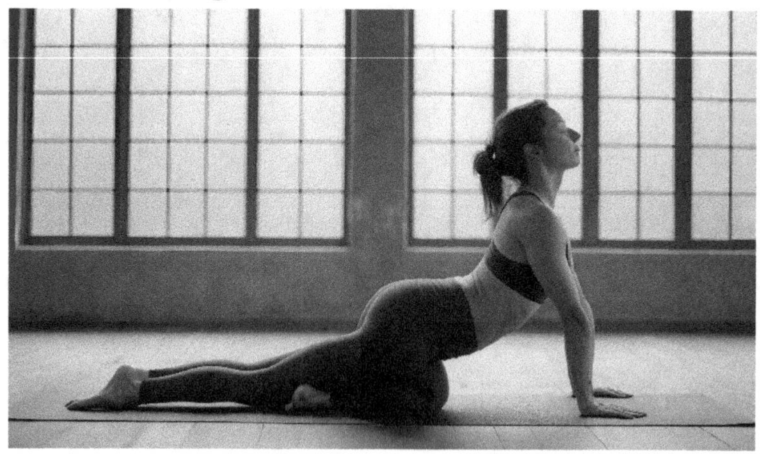

1. Warrior II (Virabhadrasana II)

Description:

1. From standing, step your feet wide apart.
2. Turn your right foot out 90 degrees and your left foot slightly inward.
3. Bend your right knee over your right ankle, extending your arms parallel to the floor, with palms facing down.
4. Gaze over your right fingertips.

- Duration: Hold for 30 seconds to 1 minute on each side.

Keep your hips squared towards the side, sinking down through the back thigh.

Engage your core and lift through the chest. Press evenly through both feet.

Benefits:

Strengthens legs, improves balance and focus, opens hips and chest.

2. Triangle Pose (Trikonasana)

Description:

1. Start in Warrior II, straighten your right leg and reach your right arm forward, then lower your right hand to your shin, ankle, or the floor.
2. Extend your left arm towards the sky, stacking shoulders.
3. Keep your torso open and gaze towards your top hand.
4.

- Duration: Hold for 30 seconds to 1 minute on each side.

Tips:

Engage your thighs and lengthen your spine.

Press into the outer edge of your back foot.

Use a block under your bottom hand if reaching the floor is challenging

.

Benefits:

Stretches hamstrings, hips, and spine, improves digestion, strengthens legs and core.

3. Half Moon Pose (Ardha Chandrasana)

Description:

1. From Triangle Pose, bend your right knee slightly and shift your weight onto your right foot.

2. Lift your left leg parallel to the floor, toes pointing towards the left.

3. Extend your left arm towards the sky, stacking shoulders. Keep your hips and chest open.

Tips:

Engage your core for stability and keep a micro-bend in your standing knee.

Use a block under your bottom hand for support if needed.

- Duration: Hold for 30 seconds to 1 minute on each side.

Benefits:

Improves balance and coordination, strengthens legs and ankles, stretches groins and hamstrings.

4. Extended Side Angle Pose (Utthita Parsvakonasana)

Description:

1. From Warrior II, lower your right hand to the inside or outside of your right foot.

2. Extend your left arm overhead, biceps by the ear, palm facing down.

3. Keep your chest open and gaze towards your top hand.

- Duration: Hold for 30 seconds to 1 minute on each side.

Tips:

Keep your right knee stacked over your ankle, and your thigh parallel to the floor.

Engage your core for stability and press into the outer edge of your back foot.

Benefits:

Strengthens legs and core, stretches groins and side body, improves balance and concentration.

5. Bridge Pose (Setu Bandhasana)

Description:

1. Lie on your back with knees bent and feet hip-width apart.
2. Press into your feet and lift your hips towards the sky, interlacing your hands beneath your back.
3. Keep your thighs parallel and press your chest towards your

- Duration: Hold for 30 seconds to 1 minute on each side.

Benefits:

Strengthens back, glutes, and hamstrings, stretches chest and shoulders, improves spine flexibility.

Tips:

Engage your glutes and thighs to lift your hips higher.

Keep your neck long and avoid collapsing into your shoulders.

You can also place a block under your sacrum for support.

6. Revolved Triangle Pose (Parivrtta Trikonasana)

Description:

1. From Warrior II, straighten your right leg and hinge at your hips to reach your right hand to the outside of your left foot.
2. Extend your left arm towards the sky, stacking shoulders.
3. Keep your chest open and gaze towards your top hand.

- Duration: Hold for 30 seconds to 1 minute on each side.

Benefits:

Stretches hamstrings, hips, and spine, improves digestion, strengthens legs and core

7. Camel Pose (Ustrasana)

Description:

1. Kneel on the mat with knees hip-width apart. Place your hands on your lower back, fingers pointing down.
2. Lean back, lifting your chest towards the sky.
3. Reach your hands towards your heels, keeping your hips stacked over knees.

- Duration: Hold for 30 seconds to 1 minute

Tips:

Press your thighs and hips forward as you lift your chest.

Keep your neck long and avoid compressing the lower back.

Engage your core for stability.

Benefits:

Stretches front body, thighs, and hip flexors, improves posture, stimulates digestion.

8. Seated Forward Bend (Paschimottanasana)

Description:

1. Sit on the mat with legs extended in front of you.
2. Inhale to lengthen your spine, then exhale to fold forward from the hips, reaching for your feet or shins.
3. Keep your spine straight and chest open.

- Duration: Hold for 30 seconds to 1 minute

Benefits:

Stretches hamstrings and spine, calms the mind, relieves stress and anxiety.

9. Plank Pose (Phalakasana)

Description:

1. Start in a high push-up position, wrists under shoulders and body in a straight line from head to heels.
2. Engage your core, quads, and glutes, pressing away from the floor.
3. Hold the position, breathing steadily.

- Duration: Hold for 30 seconds to 1 minute

Benefits:

Strengthens core, arms, and shoulders, improves posture, boosts metabolism.

10. Boat Pose (Navasana)

Description:

1. Sit on the mat with knees bent and feet flat.

Tips:

Engage your core to lift your chest and legs higher.

Keep your spine straight and lengthen through the crown of your head.

Modify by keeping your knees bent if needed.

2. Lean back slightly, lift your feet off the floor, and straighten your legs, forming a V shape with your torso and legs.

3. Extend your arms forward, parallel to the floor.

- Duration: Hold for 30 seconds to 1 minute

Benefits:

Strengthens core muscles, improves balance and stability, stimulates digestion.

11. Upward-Facing Dog Pose (Urdhva Mukha Svanasana)

Description:

4. Lie face down on the mat, palms flat near your ribs.

5. Press into your hands to lift your chest and thighs off the mat, keeping your arms straight.

Tips:

Engage your thighs and lift your kneecaps off the mat.

Keep your shoulders away from your ears and open your chest.

Modify by lowering your hips if needed.

6. Roll your shoulders back and lift your gaze towards the sky.

- Duration: Hold for 15-30 seconds.

Benefits:

Strengthens arms, wrists, and back muscles, improves posture, stretches abdomen and chest.

12. Low Lunge (Anjaneyasana)

Description:

1. From a standing position, step your right foot back into a lunge, lowering your right knee to the mat.
2. Keep your left knee over your ankle and your torso upright.
3. Raise your arms overhead, reaching towards the sky.

Engage your core and lift through your chest. Sink your hips forward and down to deepen the stretch.

Use a blanket under your knee for extra support if needed.

- Duration: Hold for 30 seconds to 1 minute on each side

Benefits:

Stretches hip flexors and quadriceps, opens chest and shoulders, improves balance.

13. Revolved Chair Pose (Parivrtta Utkatasana)

Description:

1. Begin in Chair Pose, with feet together and knees bent, as if sitting back in an invisible chair.
2. Twist your torso to the right, bringing your left elbow to the outside of your right knee.
3. Extend your right arm towards the sky, keeping your chest open.

- Duration: Hold for 30 seconds to 1 minute on each side

Benefits:

Strengthens legs, core, and spine, improves digestion, detoxifies the body.

14. Crow Pose (Bakasana)

Description:

1. Squat down with feet hip-width apart.
2. Place your hands shoulder-width apart on the mat, fingers spread wide.
3. Bend your elbows slightly and bring your knees to rest on the backs of your upper arms.
4. Shift your weight forward, lifting your feet off the mat.

Tips:

Engage your core and squeeze your inner thighs towards your torso.

Look forward and keep your gaze steady.

Start by lifting one foot at a time, then both.

- Duration: Hold for 15-30 seconds.

Benefits:

Strengthens arms, wrists, and core muscles, improves balance and focus, builds confidence.

15. Fish Pose (Matsyasana)

Description:

1. Lie on your back with legs extended and arms by your sides.
2. Press your forearms and elbows into the mat, lifting your chest towards the sky.
3. Tilt your head back and rest the crown of your head on the mat.

- Duration: Hold for 30 seconds to 1 minute.

Benefits:

Opens chest and throat, stretches neck and shoulders, stimulates thyroid and parathyroid glands.

Chapter Nine:
Yoga for Juniors

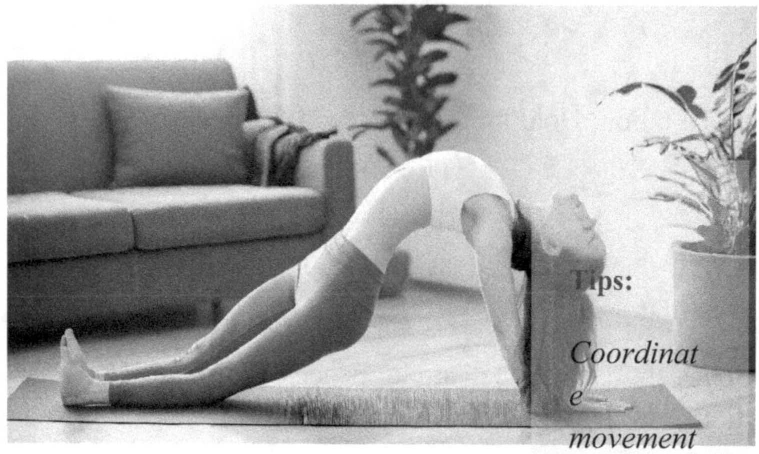

1. Cat-Cow Pose (Marjaryasana-Bitilasana)

Description:

1. Start on your hands and knees, wrists under shoulders and knees under hips.
2. Inhale, arch your back, lift your tailbone and head (Cow Pose).

3. Exhale, round your spine, tuck your chin to your chest (Cat Pose). Flow smoothly between the two poses.

- Duration: Hold each position for 5-10 breaths.

Benefits:

Warms up the spine, increases flexibility, massages internal organs.

2. Downward-Facing Dog Pose (Adho Mukha Svanasana)

Description:

1. Start on your hands and knees, then lift your hips towards the sky, straightening your arms and legs to form an inverted V shape.

Tips:

Keep a slight bend in your knees if needed.

Press into your fingertips to relieve pressure on your wrists.

Focus on lengthening your spine and reaching your tailbone towards the ceiling.

2. Press your palms into the mat and your heels towards the floor.

- Duration: Hold for 5-10 breaths.

Benefits:

Stretches shoulders, hamstrings, calves, and spine, strengthens arms and legs, improves circulation.

3. Tree Pose (Vrksasana)

Description:

1. Stand tall with feet hip-width apart.
2. Shift your weight onto your left foot and place the sole of your right foot on your inner left thigh or calf.

3. Bring your palms together at your heart center or extend your arms overhead.

- Duration: Hold for 5-10 breaths.

Benefits:

Improves balance and concentration, strengthens ankles and thighs, opens hips and chest.

4. Butterfly Pose (Baddha Konasana)

Description:

1. Sit on the mat with soles of your feet together and knees bent out to the sides.
2. Hold onto your ankles or feet with your hands.
3. Sit up tall, lengthening your spine.

Tips:

Gently press your knees towards the floor using your elbows.

Keep your shoulders relaxed and your chest open.

You can also gently flap your knees up and down like butterfly wings.

- Duration: Hold for 5-10 breaths.

Benefits:

Stretches inner thighs and groin, opens hips, improves flexibility in knees and hips.

5. Cobra Pose (Bhujangasana)

Description:

1. Lie on your stomach with palms flat near your ribs.
2. Press into your hands to lift your chest off the mat, keeping your elbows close to your body.
3. Lengthen your neck and gaze forward.

Tips:

Press the tops of your feet into the mat and engage your legs.

Use the strength of your back muscles to lift your chest, rather than relying on your hands.

Keep your shoulders away from your ears.

- Duration: Hold for 5-10 breaths.

Benefits:

Strengthens back muscles, stretches chest and abdomen, improves posture.

6. Child's Pose (Balasana)

Description:

1. Kneel on the mat with big toes touching and knees apart.
2. Lower your torso between your thighs and extend your arms forward, palms down.
3. Rest your forehead on the mat.

Tips:

Relax your shoulders and breathe deeply into your lower back.

Sink your hips towards your heels and allow your chest to melt towards the mat.

You can place a cushion under your forehead for support.

- Duration: Hold for 5-10 breaths.

Benefits:

Stretches hips, thighs, and ankles, relieves back and neck tension, calms the mind.

7. Happy Baby Pose (Ananda Balasana)

Description:

1. Lie on your back and draw your knees towards your chest.
2. Grab the outer edges of your feet with your hands, and gently open your knees wider than your torso.
3. Keep your tailbone grounded.

- Duration: Hold for 30 seconds to 1 minute.

Benefits:

Stretches groin and inner thighs, releases tension in lower back, calms the mind.

8. Upward-Facing Dog Pose (Urdhva Mukha Svanasana)

Description:

1. Lie face down on the mat, palms flat near your ribs.
2. Press into your hands to lift your chest and thighs off the mat, keeping your arms straight.
3. Roll your shoulders back and lift your gaze towards the sky.

Tips:

Engage your thighs and lift your kneecaps off the mat.

Keep your shoulders away from your ears and open your chest.

Modify by lowering your hips if needed.

- Duration: Hold for 15-30 seconds.

Benefits:

Strengthens arms, wrists, and back muscles, improves posture, stretches abdomen and chest.

9. Extended Triangle Pose (Utthita Trikonasana)

Description:

1. From a standing position, step your feet wide apart.
2. Turn your right foot out 90 degrees and your left foot slightly inward.
3. Extend your arms parallel to the floor.
4. Reach your right hand forward as you hinge at the hips and lower your right hand to your shin, ankle, or the floor.

5. Extend your left arm towards the sky, stacking shoulders.

- Duration: Hold for 30 seconds to 1 minute on each side

Benefits:

Stretches hamstrings, hips, and side body, improves balance and posture.

10. Seated Twist (Ardha Matsyendrasana)

Description:

1. Sit on the mat with legs extended in front of you.
2. Bend your right knee and place your right foot outside your left thigh.
3. Hug your right knee with your left arm.
4. Inhale, lengthen your spine, then exhale and twist to the right, bringing your right hand behind you.

Tips:

Keep both sit bones grounded.

Lengthen your spine with each inhale and deepen the twist with each exhale.

Gaze over your right shoulder.

- Duration: Hold for 30 seconds to 1 minute on each side

Benefits:

Improves digestion, massages abdominal organs, stretches spine and shoulders.

11. Warrior I Pose (Virabhadrasana I)

Description:

1. From standing, step your left foot back and angle it slightly out.
2. Bend your right knee over your ankle as you square your hips forward.
3. Extend your arms overhead, palms facing each other.

- Duration: Hold for 30 seconds to 1 minute on each side

Benefits:

Strengthens legs, opens hips and chest, builds concentration and focus.

12. Extended Puppy Pose (Uttana Shishosana)

Description:

1. Start on your hands and knees, then walk your hands forward as you lower your chest towards the mat, keeping your hips stacked over your knees.
2. Rest your forehead on the mat and extend your arms forward.

Press into your palms to lift your armpits away from the floor.

Keep your hips above your knees and lengthen through your spine.

Relax your neck and breathe deeply.

- Duration: Hold for 30 seconds to 1 minute.

Benefits:

Stretches spine, shoulders, and arms, calms the mind, relieves tension in upper body.

13. Standing Forward Bend (Uttanasana)

Description:

1. From a standing position, hinge at your hips and fold forward, bringing your chest towards your thighs and your hands towards the floor or legs.
2. Keep your spine straight and lengthen through the crown of your head.

- Duration: Hold for 30 seconds to 1 minute.

Benefits:

Stretches hamstrings and spine, calms the mind, relieves stress and anxiety.

14. Garland Pose (Malasana)

Description:

1. Start in a squat position with feet wider than hip-width apart, toes turned out.
2. Lower your hips towards the floor, bringing your elbows to the inside of your knees.
3. Bring your palms together at heart center, pressing your elbows against your inner thighs.

Tips:

Keep your chest lifted and spine long.

Engage your core to support your lower back.

Use a block under your heels if needed for support.

- Duration: Hold for 30 seconds to 1 minute.

Benefits:

Stretches ankles, groin, and lower back, improves digestion, strengthens core and legs.

15.Corpse Pose (Savasana)

Description:

1. Lie on your back with legs extended and arms by your sides, palms facing up.
2. Close your eyes and allow your body to completely relax into the mat.

- Duration: Remain in Savasana for 5-10 minutes.

Benefits:

Relaxes the body and mind, reduces stress and anxiety, improves concentration and sleep quality.

Chapter Ten:
Yoga for Seniors

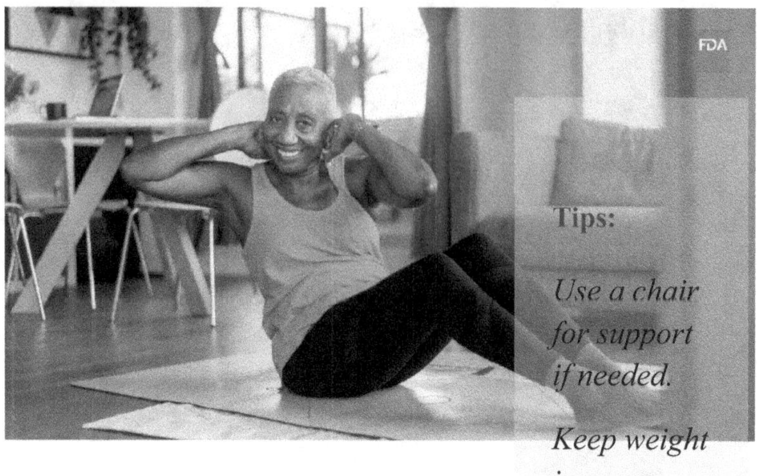

1. Chair Pose (Utkatasana)

Description:

1. Begin by standing with feet hip-width apart. Inhale and raise arms overhead, palms facing each other.
2. Exhale and bend your knees, lowering your hips as if sitting back into a chair.

3. Keep your chest lifted and gaze forward.

- Duration: Hold for 15-30 seconds.

Benefits:

Strengthens legs and core, improves balance, increases mobility in hips and knees.

2. Tree Pose (Vrikshasana)

Description:

1. Stand tall with feet hip-width apart.
2. Shift weight onto your left foot and place the sole of your right foot on your inner left thigh or calf.
3. Bring hands to heart center or extend arms overhead.

Tips:

Use a wall or chair for support if needed.

Focus on a point in front of you for balance.

Avoid placing foot on the knee to protect joints.

- Duration: Hold for 15-30 seconds on each side.

Benefits:

Improves balance, strengthens ankles and legs, increases focus and concentration.

3. Seated Forward Bend (Paschimottanasana)

Description:

1. Sit on the floor with legs extended in front of you.
2. Inhale to lengthen the spine, then exhale to hinge at the hips and fold forward.
3. Reach for your feet or shins, keeping spine straight.

- Duration: Hold for 15-30 seconds.

Benefits:

Stretches spine, hamstrings, and calves, relieves tension in lower back, calms the mind.

4. Supported Bridge Pose

Description:

1. Lie on your back with knees bent and feet hip-width apart.
2. Place a block under your sacrum and relax onto it.
3. Keep arms by your sides with palms facing up.

Tips:

Adjust block height as needed for comfort.

Relax into the pose and focus on deep breathing.

Engage pelvic floor muscles gently.

- Duration: Hold for 30-60 seconds.

Benefits:

Stretches chest and shoulders, relieves back pain, reduces stress and anxiety.

5. Legs-Up-the-Wall Pose (Viparita Karani)

Description:

1. Sit with your side against a wall.
2. Lie back and swing your legs up the wall, keeping hips close to the wall.
3. Relax arms by your sides, palms facing up.

Tips:

Use a folded blanket or cushion under hips for support if needed.

Keep legs straight or slightly bent.

Close eyes and focus on deep breathing.

- Duration: Hold for 3-5 minutes.

Benefits:

Improves circulation, reduces swelling in legs and feet, relaxes nervous system.

6. Mountain Pose (Tadasana)

Description:

1. Stand tall with feet hip-width apart, arms by your sides.
2. Press feet into the ground and reach crown of head towards the sky.
3. Relax shoulders down and back.

Tips:

Engage thigh muscles and lift arches of feet.

Keep spine long and breathe deeply.

Imagine roots growing from feet into the earth.

- Duration: Hold for 30-60 seconds.

Benefits:

Improves posture, strengthens legs and feet, increases energy and focus.

7. Warrior I (Virabhadrasana I)

Description:

1. From standing, step your right foot back and turn it out slightly.
2. Bend your left knee, stacking it over the ankle.
3. Reach arms overhead with palms facing each other. Square hips forward.

Tips:

Keep back leg straight and grounded.

Engage core muscles for stability.

Gaze forward or up between hands.

- Duration: Hold for 15-30 seconds on each side.

Benefits:

Strengthens legs and core, opens hips and chest, builds confidence and courage.

8. Warrior II (Virabhadrasana II)

Description:

1. From Warrior I, open hips and arms to the sides, parallel to the floor.
2. Keep front knee bent, pointing over toes.
3. Gaze over front fingertips.

Tips:

Keep shoulders relaxed and chest open.

Press into outer edge of back foot.

Sink hips low but keep spine long.

- Duration: Hold for 15-30 seconds on each side.

Benefits:

Improves balance and stability, strengthens legs and core, increases focus and concentration.

9. Corpse Pose (Savasana)

Description:

1. Lie on your back with legs extended and arms by your sides, palms facing up.
2. Close your eyes and relax your entire body, allowing it to melt into the floor.

- Duration: Hold for 5-10 minutes.

Benefits:

Reduces stress and anxiety, promotes relaxation and better sleep, integrates the benefits of practice.

10. Seated Cat-Cow Stretch

Description:

1. Sit comfortably in a chair with feet flat on the floor.
2. Inhale, arch your back, and lift your chest (Cow Pose).
3. Exhale, round your spine, and tuck your chin to your chest (Cat Pose).
4. Repeat slowly, coordinating movement with breath.

Tips:

Move gently and smoothly, focusing on spinal mobility.

Keep your shoulders relaxed and breathe deeply into each movement.

- Duration: Repeat 5-10 times.

Benefits:

Improves flexibility and mobility in the spine, relieves back pain, massages internal organs.

11.Chair Yoga Twist

Description:

1. Sit sideways on a chair with feet flat on the floor. Hold the backrest with both hands for support.
2. Inhale, lengthen your spine, and exhale, twist gently towards the back of the chair.
3. Hold for a few breaths, then repeat on the other side.

- Duration: Hold for 30 seconds to 1 minute on each side.

Benefits:

Improves spinal mobility, stimulates digestion, releases tension in the back and hips

12. Legs-Up-the-Wall Pose (Viparita Karani)

Description:

1. Sit sideways on the floor next to a wall.
2. Lie on your back and swing your legs up against the wall, keeping your hips close to the wall.
3. Rest your arms by your sides with palms facing up. Relax and breathe deeply.

- Duration: Hold for 5-10 minutes.

Benefits:

Relieves swelling in the legs and feet, reduces stress and anxiety, promotes relaxation and better sleep.

13. Seated Spinal Twist

Description:

1. Sit on a chair with feet flat on the floor.
2. Inhale, lengthen your spine, then exhale, twist gently to the right, placing your left hand on the outside of your right knee and your right hand on the back of the chair.
3. Hold for a few breaths, then switch sides.

- Duration: Hold for 30 seconds to 1 minute on each side.

Benefits:

Improves spinal mobility, stimulates digestion, relieves tension in the back and shoulders.

14. Seated Side Stretch

Description:

1. Sit on a chair with feet flat on the floor.
2. Inhale, raise your right arm overhead, and lean to the left, stretching the right side of your body.
3. Hold for a few breaths, then switch sides.

Tips:

Keep your shoulders relaxed and your spine tall.

Engage your core to support the stretch and avoid collapsing into the side body.

- Duration: Hold for 30 seconds to 1 minute on each side.

Benefits:

Stretches the side body, opens the lungs for deeper breathing, improves posture.

15. Seated Wide-Legged Forward Bend

Description:

1. Sit on the edge of a chair with legs extended wide apart.
2. Inhale, lengthen your spine, then exhale, hinge forward from your hips, reaching for the floor or your feet.
3. Keep your back flat and chest open.

- Duration: Hold for 30 seconds to 1 minute.

Benefits:

Stretches the inner thighs and hamstrings, stimulates the abdominal organs, relieves tension in the back and hips

16. Chair Supported Shoulderstand

Description:

1. Sit comfortably in a chair with your back against the backrest.
2. Lift your legs up towards the ceiling, resting them against the wall.
3. Support your lower back with your hands on the seat of the chair.

Tips:

Keep your neck and head in line with your spine.

Press your shoulders down away from your ears and engage your core for stability.

- Duration: Hold for 1-2 minutes.

Benefits:

Improves circulation, reduces swelling in the legs and feet, relieves back tension.

17. Reclining Bound Angle Pose (Supta Baddha Konasana)

Description:

1. Lie on your back with knees bent and feet flat on the floor.
2. Let your knees fall open to the sides and bring the soles of your feet together.
3. Support your knees with cushions or blocks if needed.

- Duration: Hold for 1-5 minutes.

Benefits:

Stretches the inner thighs and groin, opens the hips and pelvis, promotes relaxation and stress relief.

18. Seated Eagle Arms

Description:

1. Sit comfortably in a chair with feet flat on the floor.
2. Extend your arms forward at shoulder height, then cross your right arm over your left, wrapping your forearms and pressing your palms together.

- Duration: Hold for 30 seconds to 1 minute, then switch sides.

Benefits:

Releases tension in the upper back and shoulders, improves posture, increases circulation to the arms and hands.

19. Supine Spinal Twist

Description:

1. Lie on your back with knees bent and feet flat on the floor.
2. Extend your arms out to the sides in line with your shoulders.
3. Exhale, lower your knees to the right side, keeping both shoulders grounded.

Tips:

Keep your knees stacked and your spine aligned.

Turn your head to the opposite side for a deeper stretch.

Breathe deeply into the twist.

- Duration: Hold for 30 seconds
  to 1 minute on each side.

Benefits:

Improves spinal mobility, releases
tension in the back and hips,
massages internal organs.

20. Corpse Pose (Savasana)

Description:

1. Lie on your back with legs
   extended and arms by
   your sides, palms facing
   up.
2. Close your eyes and relax
   your entire body, letting
   go of any tension or effort.
3. Breathe naturally and
   allow your mind to
   become still.

Tips:

Make yourself comfortabl e with cushions or blankets under your head, neck, and knees.

Let go of any thoughts and simply surrender to the present moment.

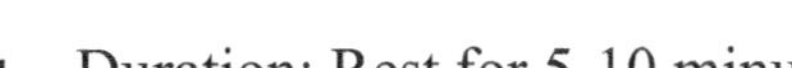

- Duration: Rest for 5-10 minutes.

Benefits:

Promotes deep relaxation and stress relief, rejuvenates the body and mind, integrates the benefits of the practice.

Conclusion

Congratulations on completing this journey through the world of yoga! By now, you've experienced the numerous physical, mental, and emotional benefits that yoga has to offer. But your journey doesn't end here. In this final chapter, let's explore how you can integrate yoga into your daily life and continue your yoga journey for lifelong well-being.

Integrating Yoga into Your Daily Life:

1. Set Realistic Goals: Reflect on your yoga journey and set realistic goals for yourself. Whether it's practicing yoga for a certain number of days per week, mastering a challenging pose, or simply finding moments of stillness and mindfulness each day, set intentions that align with your lifestyle and priorities.

2. Create a Routine: Establishing a consistent yoga practice is key to reaping its benefits. Schedule regular times for yoga practice each day or week, whether it's in the morning to energize your day, during a lunch break to recharge, or in the evening to unwind and relax.

3. Start Small: Remember that even a short yoga practice can make a significant difference. If time is limited, commit to just a few minutes of yoga each day. Whether it's a few sun salutations, a brief meditation, or a gentle stretch, every bit counts towards your well-being.

4. Incorporate Mindfulness: Yoga is not just about the physical postures; it's also about cultivating mindfulness and awareness. Bring the principles of yoga off the mat and into your daily life by practicing mindfulness in everyday activities such as eating, walking, or interacting with others.

5. **Listen to Your Body:** Honor your body's needs and limitations as you practice yoga. Be mindful of any discomfort or pain, and modify poses as needed to ensure safety and comfort. Remember that yoga is a personal journey, and it's okay to adapt your practice to suit your individual needs.

6. **Stay Consistent:** Consistency is key to progress in yoga. Even on days when you don't feel motivated to practice, show up on your mat and trust the process. Over time, you'll build strength, flexibility, and resilience both on and off the mat.

Continuing Your Yoga Journey:

1. **Explore New Styles:** Yoga offers a rich styles and traditions to explore. Whether you're drawn to the dynamic flow of vinyasa, the precision of Iyengar, the introspection of yin, or the spiritual depth of Kundalini, continue to explore and experiment with different styles to deepen your practice.

2. Attend Workshops and Retreats: Immerse yourself in the world of yoga by attending workshops, retreats, and special events. These opportunities provide valuable insights, inspiration, and connection with like-minded practitioners, teachers, and experts in the field.

3. Deepen Your Knowledge: Expand your understanding of yoga philosophy, anatomy, meditation, and breath work through further study and education. Dive into books, online courses, podcasts, and lectures to deepen your knowledge and enrich your practice.

4. **Connect with Community:** Cultivate a sense of community and support by joining yoga classes, groups, or online communities. Surround yourself with fellow yogis who inspire and encourage you on your journey, and share your experiences, challenges, and triumphs along the way.

5. **Stay Open and Curious:** Approach your yoga journey with an open mind and a sense of curiosity. Embrace the process of growth and transformation, and remain receptive

to new experiences, insights, and possibilities that arise along the way.

Remember that yoga is a lifelong journey of self-discovery, self-care, and self-realization. As you integrate yoga into your daily life and continue your journey, may you find peace, balance, and fulfillment in every breath, every posture, and every moment on and off the mat.